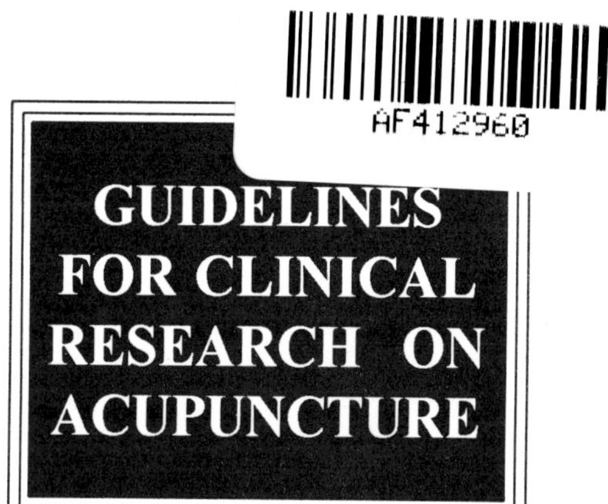


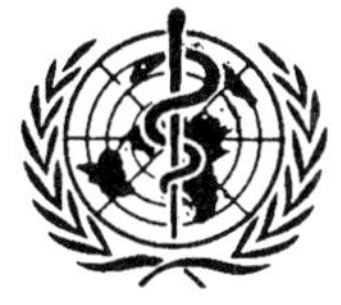

**WORLD HEALTH ORGANIZATION**
**Regional Office for the Western Pacific**
**1995**

**WHO Library Cataloguing in Publication Data**

1.      Acupuncture
2.      Research
3.      Guidelines
I.      Series

ISBN 92 9061 114 6      (NLM Classification WB 369)

# CONTENTS

# FOREWORD

Acupuncture has been widely recognized as a valuable and readily available means of health care. It is effective, requires only simple equipment and is inexpensive. However, the practice of acupuncture is still mainly based on tradition and personal experience.

Clinical studies and related research on acupuncture have been undertaken by independent groups, but the quality of research still varies considerably. The need for basic principles which can be followed by researchers involved in clinical research on acupuncture has been raised on several occasions.

In June 1994, a Working Group organized by the WHO Regional Office for the Western Pacific met in Aomori, Japan to develop guidelines for clinical research on acupuncture. This represented efforts to introduce basic principles and methods used in modern scientific research to evaluate the effectiveness of acupuncture, whilst remaining sensitive to the different nature of the discipline.

The task of developing guidelines for clinical research on acupuncture was not an easy one. The guidelines had to incorporate a broad range of issues and disciplines involved in clinical research on acupuncture. They had to be suitable for use by researchers engaged in many different areas related to the evaluation of acupuncture's effectiveness in treating various diseases and disorders. They needed to be acceptable to both traditional and modern medical disciplines.

It is hoped that these guidelines provide detailed criteria and methods which will be easily followed by researchers to design, conduct and evaluate their research project on acupuncture. However, they are also intended to be general enough to enable researchers to modify them to suit their own specific needs.

The publication of these guidelines will definitely promote clinical research on acupuncture in the Region as well as in other parts of the world. Although the experience obtained through the use of acupuncture over many years should not be ignored, scientific research on acupuncture will provide additional evidence to reconfirm its effectiveness, thereby enhancing its acceptance and utilization.

**S.T. Han, MD, Ph. D.**
**Regional Director**

# 1.   INTRODUCTION

## Background

Acupuncture has been applied as a therapeutic medical technique in China for more than 2500 years although its development goes back further than that. In the 2nd and 3rd century BC, the systematical theory of acupuncture was already well developed as shown in the Huang Di Nei Jing (The Yellow Emperor's Internal Classic). Acupuncture, as an apparently simple and effective clinical procedure, was introduced to China's neighbouring countries, Korea, Japan and Viet Nam, in the 6th century. In the early 16th century, acupuncture came to Europe.

During the last two decades, acupuncture has spread worldwide. There has been growing interest in the therapeutic applications of acupuncture, and a desire to explain its modes of action in terms of modern scientific knowledge. WHO has been aware of the potential value of acupuncture and its possible contribution to WHO's goal of health for all. In 1985, the Regional Committee for the Western Pacific adopted a resolution on traditional medicine which recognized that traditional medicine practices, particularly those of herbal medicine and acupuncture, constitute appropriate technologies which could be integrated into the national health strategies, and urged Member States to initiate programmes of research, training and information. Two years later, in 1987, another resolution was adopted by the Regional Committee, reiterating the value of herbal medicine and acupuncture and urging Member States to establish or further develop programmes on traditional medicine, particularly herbal and acupuncture, in the light of their specific needs and circumstances.

## Research on acupuncture

Acupuncture is recognized as a valuable and readily available resource for health care throughout the world. However, the use of acupuncture is based mainly on traditional and personal experience. Although acupuncture has been tested by thousands of years of clinical practice, appropriate scientific studies would now be useful for the rational use and further development of acupuncture. The need for further clinical research does not challenge the widespread acceptance of acupuncture.

Two resolutions concerning traditional medicine adopted by the WHO Regional Committee for the Western Pacific encouraged Member States to undertake research on evaluating the safety and efficacy of traditional medicine (acupuncture and herbal medicine), based on the concepts of both modern and traditional medicine.

Research on evaluating the clinical effectiveness of acupuncture should be given more emphasis than investigating the mechanism of its therapeutic effect, as the former is directly concerned with the promotion and delivery of acupuncture in health care services.

## Need for guidelines for the clinical evaluation of acupuncture

Clinical studies and related research have been undertaken by independent groups, but the quality of research varies considerably. Acceptable results should be brought together for comparison and conclusions. It has proved difficult to apply and integrate the basic principles and methodology of modern science that ensure the reliability of research subjects to clinical studies on acupuncture. Application of basic principles and methodology of modern science, i.e. design, conduct, statistical analysis, interpretation and reporting, were not properly understood by acupuncture researchers. In 1989, a WHO scientific group which met in Geneva recommended that WHO play a role in consolidating guidelines on research methodology so as to ensure the acceptable quality of results.

# 2.  GLOSSARY

The terms below are used as working definitions in this document.

## Terms relating to evaluation methodology

1.  Validity - Validity is the degree to which the result of measurement corresponds with the true state of the phenomenon to be measured. There are two general kinds of validity:

    - internal validity, the degree to which the results of an observation are correct for the patients to be studied; and

    - external validity, the degree to which the results of an observation hold true in other settings. Generalizability is the other word for external validity.

2.  Reliability - Reliability is the extent to which repeated measurements of a relatively stable phenomenon fall closely together. Reproducibility and precision are other words for this property.

3.  Statistical significance (P-value) - A value associated with an observed test statistic that indicates the probability that a value is as extreme or more extreme than the one observed will arise by chance alone in repeated replications of a study.

## Terms relating specifically to acupuncture studies

1.  Acupuncture - Involves the act of needle insertion, although there are many other non-invasive techniques for acupuncture point stimulation. Points may be selected according to:

    - traditional medical systems;

- symptoms;

- point selection based on the scientific relationships of point function; and

- point prescription.

2. Real acupuncture - Acupuncture given as a real clinical treatment.

3. Sham acupuncture - Inappropriate acupuncture for the condition being treated taking into account the acupuncture microsystem.

4. Mock Transcutaneous Electrical Nerve Stimulation - Treatment with a defunctioned TENS machine in which no electrical stimulus reaches the patient but the TENS machine appears to be active.

5. Minimal acupuncture - Shallow needle insertion which in some studies has been used as a placebo, but in others as real treatment.

6. Control group - A comparative group with which to compare the effects of real acupuncture treatment. The control group might be untreated or receive conventional medical treatment.

7. Placebo - If acupuncture is defined as skin penetration with an acupuncture needle, then true placebo acupuncture would appear to be impossible. Less effective forms of acupuncture can be perfectly adequate controls, and in some specific instances it may be possible to mimic acupuncture in a credible manner.

# 3. GOALS AND OBJECTIVES OF THE GUIDELINES

## Goals

- To strengthen clinical research on acupuncture.

- To promote the rational use of acupuncture.

## Objectives

- To provide basic principles and applicable standards for researchers and acupuncture practitioners to prepare and conduct clinical evaluation on the effectiveness of acupuncture.

- To provide basic criteria for peer review and monitoring research proposals as well as implement the results of the research.

- To facilitate the exchange of research experience and other information so that a body of reliable data for the validation of acupuncture can be accumulated.

- To provide criteria for interested policy-makers to select and determine the application of acupuncture.

# 4.  GENERAL CONSIDERATIONS

## Legal considerations

Governments should actively encourage research on acupuncture, particularly clinical evaluation, as well-designed research will provide reliable references regarding the validity of acupuncture practice.

Legislation on acupuncture and regulation of acupuncture practice can play an important role in assuring the quality of acupuncture service and administration of acupuncture practice.

## Ethical considerations

Clinical research on acupuncture must be carried out in accordance with all four relevant ethical principles: justice, respect for persons, beneficence and non-maleficence.  If animals are used their welfare must be respected.

## Considering the character of acupuncture

Acupuncture was developed as a branch of traditional Chinese medicine on the basis of oriental philosophy which takes a holistic approach to regulating the balance of the human body. (Several different schools of acupuncture exist each with its own principles.)  Respect for these principles must be an important priority in any research on this topic. These principles may vary with the types of acupuncture being investigated. To this end traditional knowledge and experience of acupuncture should be duly represented on the investigative team when research is proposed, prepared and conducted.

A good clinical study on acupuncture should be conducted with the understanding and integration of both traditional and/or modern knowledge of medicine. Criteria for diagnosis of both traditional and modern medicine may be used.

# Clinical research

## Aims

Acupuncture may be used as:

1.      a therapeutic intervention including rehabilitation; and

2.      a preventive and health maintenance intervention.

In this context, clinical research in acupuncture may be conducted to help guide:

1.      practitioners in their choice of treatment;

2.      the patient in deciding whether to choose acupuncture as a mode of treatment; and

3.      health care policy-makers in their decisions.

Clinical research in acupuncture may also benefit other health professionals and the scientific community, as research in acupuncture may provide important heuristics for their works.

## Selection of research projects

Research projects should be selected with due consideration for several factors in addition to scientific interest, such as the potential value of research results for improving the health of the community, with regard to the local prevalence of disease. The scientific acceptability of the project and the feasibility of using alternatives should be considered. An evaluation may be carried out to provide new scientific evidence for traditional experience. It may also be conducted to validate new indications of acupuncture points or new combinations of points. A comparative study on the effectiveness of different points or groups of points may also be conducted. Various needling techniques may be analysed to compare their efficacy.

## Laboratory studies

Related laboratory studies on acupuncture will provide useful ideas and serve as reference when clinical research on acupuncture is prepared or conducted.

## Animal research

Animal research may be conducted for the purpose of (a) veterinary treatment and (b) basic research. There are some situations in which animal experiments are not relevant to the human situation.

## Education

Dissemination of knowledge about acupuncture and acupuncture research to professional health workers in the form of courses can greatly aid the overall efforts to improve the clinical evaluation of acupuncture.

The general public will also benefit from adequate information on the clinical effects of acupuncture and the outcome of clinical research.

# 5.  RESEARCH METHODOLOGY

## Literature review

As acupuncture was developed before the advent of modern science and is based on a different culture and philosophy, and has only recently been investigated scientifically, it must be recognized that knowledge about acupuncture is to be found in anecdotal observations rather than in systematic laboratory and clinical studies that have been published in the scientific literature.  Furthermore, it must also be recognized that while some publications on acupuncture may not meet the stringent requirements of international peer-reviewed journals, but they may still provide potentially useful observations and ideas for further study.  Therefore, a thorough literature survey should be the starting point for the clinical evaluation of acupuncture.

## Terminology and technology

To ensure the reproducibility of a clinical study on acupuncture, related terminology and technology should be clearly presented and exact protocols should be established.

- Standard acupuncture nomenclature.  The standard acupuncture nomenclature developed by the WHO Regional Office for the Western Pacific and recommended by a WHO scientific group that met in Geneva in 1989 should be used during the study.

- Length and diameter of needle(s) should be given in mm.

- Considering the lack of international standards for the location of acupuncture points, the way to locate point(s) clinically should be described and used by all investigators involved in the study.  The use of anatomical marks on the body for locating point(s) should be encouraged.

- Needling techniques of inserting, retaining, stimulating and withdrawing, should be standardized and stated in the protocol. All efforts for limiting the individual influence of investigators on the performance of the needling technique should be considered.

- The use of auxiliary acupuncture equipment such as lasers or electrical stimulators should be clearly described.

- Other factors related to the patient's condition may also need to be reported such as biorhythm, breathing and position.

## Investigators

- The investigators are responsible for the trial and for the rights, health and welfare of the subjects in the trial.

- All investigators and health providers involved in the study should have appropriate expertise, qualifications and competence to undertake a proposed study. It is recommended that a team be organized which includes acupuncture practitioners and professional health workers, as knowledge of both acupuncture and the special field for which the effectiveness of acupuncture will be evaluated will be needed for preparing and conducting a reliable clinical study.

- The investigative group must be aware of the following responsibilities:

  1. appropriate and ongoing care of patients in the study;

  2. ethical requirements for the study (for instance the need to terminate protocol treatment if the patient appears to be harmed by the continuation of the study);

  3. knowledge of acupuncture; and

  4. an appreciation of research methodology.

# Clinical research design and rational use of acupuncture

Clinical research is carried out to allow:

1.	the patient to receive more information about treatment;

2.	the practitioner to make clearer decisions about treatment options;

3.	health policy and funding authorities to make appropriate decisions about utility and cost-effectiveness.

The purpose of clinical acupuncture research is therefore:

1.	to allow the patient to make decisions based on:

- effectiveness (absolute and relative)

- safety

- cost

- relationship with intercurrent conventional care

- cultural factors and patient preference; and

2.	to develop guidelines for good clinical practice for acupuncturists.

A similar agenda exists for both the practitioner and the health funding organization.

This should lead to the rational use of acupuncture.

The methods of clinical research available to us include:

- randomized controlled clinical trials;

- cohort studies;

- retrospective studies/case control studies;

- outcome research;

- sequential trial design;

- single patient studies;

- clinical audit;

- acupuncture epidemiology;

- anthropological studies; and

- post-marketing surveillance.

A clinical trial is defined as a scientific experiment involving human subjects in which treatment is initiated for therapy evaluation.

The conduct of clinical trials is governed by the underlying purpose of the study and is therefore directly related to the outcome. A clinical trial has three fundamental components:

1. Input. This includes the patients entered, the people involved in study design and provision of therapy, data collection systems and treatment.

2. Evaluation mechanism (design), such as randomized controlled trials (RCTs), cohort studies, case control studies and clinical audits.

3. Outcome. When outcome is used as a measurement for evaluation purposes, it is usually called "endpoint". The validity and reliability of endpoints always have to be considered. It may vary from "hard" (such as laboratory test) to "soft"(such as quality of life). The study of cost-effectiveness and cost-utility will be conducted utilizing these data.

RCTs as a "gold standard" in various methods of clinical trial, can be used to answer questions about most clinical problems. However, this approach is not always a practical and cost-effective solution. Pragmatic solutions that do not "unpack" all the treatment options may therefore be required. RCTs are open to error; for instance, patient preference may have an effect on outcome as may certain cultural environments.

Clinical audit may allow developmental research directed at identifying patients who can be helped swiftly, those whose condition can be maintained with acupuncture and those whose chronic problems can be contained to avoid potentially damaging adverse reactions from invasive conventional intervention.

# Randomized controlled clinical trial design

A randomized clinical study on acupuncture should be designed by the investigators with the involvement of a biostatistician to ensure the quality of the study.

## Selection of the patient

The patients included in the study should represent the future group of patients to whom the findings of the study will be applied. The illness should be defined exactly. The source of patients recruited, and the criteria for patients' inclusion and exclusion, should be considered carefully and stated in the protocol.

If, in the proposed study, acupuncture will be used based on a knowledge of traditional diagnosis, the patients should be selected according to diagnosis and differentiation of syndromes within traditional medicine. This should also be stated in the protocol.

## Size of the study

The size of the study should be decided according to the requirements of accepted statistical analysis. Sufficient sample size will be needed in order to provide adequate statistical power to detect a clinically significant difference between two treatment groups.

## Site(s) of investigation

Clinical research must be carried out under conditions which ensure adequate safety for the subjects. The site selected for the clinical research must have adequate facilities, including laboratories and equipment, where necessary, and sufficient clerical, medical and allied health workers to support the study as required.

Facilities should be available to meet possible emergencies.

A multicentre study may be necessary, and this may require a special administrative system to ensure that the study is conducted simultaneously and adequately at different sites by several investigators following the same protocol. The training of investigators from different sites to follow the same protocol and standardization of methods for selection of patients, termination of participation, administration, data collection and evaluation will be necessary.

## Blind techniques

Blind techniques can be used in randomized controlled clinical trials. Blinding techniques may apply to patients, investigators and outcome assessor. Whenever possible, the patient should not be aware to which treatment group which he or she has been allocated. It is difficult for the investigator who gives acupuncture to the patient to be unaware of the treatment. It is essential that assessment should be made blind to treatment. The assessor should be responsible for practitioner and recording the details of reactions and results of the treatment received by patients. It is acknowledged that an unblinded therapist may affect the patient's response.

## Randomization

In clinical trials, there are two meanings of randomization. One is random sampling of the study population from the parent population. The other is random allocation which assigns the patient to one of the treatment groups by using a chance mechanism.

A randomized controlled (clinical) trial (RCT) is a study method which uses a random allocation method. Using this method comparability of groups will be maintained. Although an RCT is the most powerful method of reducing bias in the comparative evaluation of treatment options, it may become impractical when recruiting patients to some studies in the field of acupuncture, particularly when the patient has a strong preference for acupuncture treatment. In other words, the randomization mechanism may affect the outcome both positively and negatively.

## Control groups

RCTs require one or more control groups for purposes of comparison. The control group may be (not in order of priority):

- mock TENS;

- sham acupuncture;

- non-treatment;

- standard therapy;

- real acupuncture; and

- minimal acupuncture.

The selection of the control group depends on the hypothesis being tested.

## Crossover

Crossover studies are usually inappropriate in acupuncture. In acute self-limiting conditions, the natural resolution of the illness confounds the concept of crossover technology. In chronic conditions acupuncture may work for a variable time after completion of treatment (days or years). A very prolonged washout period is required if a crossover model is to be adopted and this in itself poses ethical problems.

## Strategic approaches to randomized controlled clinical trials

There are no established rules for systematically choosing the most appropriate controls in RCTs. The currently available scientific evidence suggests that the closer one gets to a purely endorphin-mediated effect, the less relevant it is to think in terms of point location and the more misleading a real versus sham comparison may be within an RCT. Conversely, the more that acupuncture treatment is autonomically mediated, such as in the management of non-painful conditions, the more relevant it may be to use a sham versus real acupuncture model when evaluating its clinical effectiveness (see Annex 1).

## Protocol development

A protocol is a document which states the background, rationale and objectives of a trial and describes its design, methodology and organization, including statistical considerations, and the conditions under which it is to be performed and managed.  The protocol should be developed by the joint effort of representatives from several disciplines including research subjects (if possible), health workers, acupuncturists and biostatisticians. The protocol should include the following:

1. the title of the clinical study;

2. a clear statement of the objectives and purpose of the study;

3. the justification of the proposed study based on the available information including a consideration of the data on the subject from modern as well as traditional literature;

4. site and the facilities where studies will be undertaken;

5. name, address and qualifications of each investigator;

6. the type of study (e.g. controlled, open) and trial design (parallel groups, randomization (methods and procedures);

7. entry and exclusion criteria for study subjects (which may be based on diagnostic criteria of either modern or traditional medicine);

8. number of study subjects needed to achieve the study objective, based on statistical considerations;

9.     the subjective and objective clinical observations and laboratory tests which will be recorded during the course of the study;

10.     acupuncture point(s) selected for the study, justification of selection of point(s) (departures from traditional and/or modern diagnostic acupuncture techniques) and description of the way to locate the point(s) in the clinic;

11.     needle(s) and size(s) used in the study;

12.     needling technique including direction, angle and depth for inserting needle(s), retaining time, positioning of the patient and stimulation such as rolling, raising and thrusting, frequency and range, and other supplementary stimulation (reducing or reinforcing) and De Qi. If electric stimulation is used, describe the model of machines, manufacturer, type of wave form, pulse duration, voltage, or current of stimulus, frequency and polarity of electric stimulation used for the study;

13.     recording of adverse reactions;

14.     control groups to be used;

15.     schedule of treatment, treatment period and time;

16.     criteria for other treatment that may or may not be given to subjects during the study;

17.     methods of recording responses, methods of measurement, times of measurements and follow-up procedures;

18.     methodology of the evaluation of results (e.g. statistical methods and reports on patients/participants who withdraw from the study);

19.     information to be given to study subjects;

20.     information to be given to the staff involved in the study;

21.     time schedule for completion of the study;

22.    medical care to be made available to patients during or after the study that if necessary may override protocol treatment;

23.    ethical considerations and measures relating to the study;

24.    relevant communications with appropriate regulatory authorities; and

25.    list of literature referred to in the protocol.


## Research knowledge

1.    Databases on acupuncture have a cultural basis but form the essential first step of any research project. Learning from previous work is an inherent part of the scientific process and that database can provide suitable reference for published work.

2.    Descriptive research outlines the observed and uncontrolled effects of acupuncture with respect to:

- traditional Chinese medicine and its variations;

- the cultural aspects of each country's medical system;

- the process or technique of the acupuncture utilized; and

- outcomes (objective and subjective).

A descriptive study could be used as the basis for more detailed investigations.

3.    Randomized controlled clinical trials. Related problems and difficulties are outlined elsewhere.

New research strategies based on a realistic assessment of the cost and the cultural and political environments in which health care operates need consideration. These include:

a.    pragmatic research that compares outcomes from patients receiving different treatment "packages" (conventional and traditional); and

b. developmental research that allows us to develop a better understanding of cost and cost-effectiveness.

## Cohort studies

Cohort studies are essentially uncontrolled prospective investigations in which detailed data are kept and then analysed to evaluate the effects of acupuncture. The advantages of cohort studies are that they allow the researcher to formulate a coherent database upon which more detailed clinical trials can be conducted. However, too often, the protocol for these studies is poorly formulated and the data collection is incomplete and inadequate. They represent an important first step in a multimodal research approach to acupuncture. Nevertheless, the conclusions generated by such evaluation must be treated with caution until they can be confirmed with further appropriate research. For instance, they can provide information about which types of patients are likely to respond best to acupuncture for a particular condition. This helps a researcher decide on the criteria for entry into an RCT, but cohort studies, however rigorously constructed, do not prove the value of acupuncture.

## Retrospective studies/case control studies

For the purpose of this chapter, retrospective studies will refer to retrospective observations limited to a relatively small number of patients.

Retrospective research is valuable in that it may provide preliminary data on the effectiveness of a particular treatment. The difficulties usually encountered relate to the fact that often relevant data have not been collected consistently and are therefore not available to allow for proper statistical analysis. Also, proper control groups are usually not available although the limitation may be partially compensated by the use of historical matched controls. In addition, the small number of observations may reflect spurious effects rather than generalizable phenomena. The most common retrospective studies are the case control studies in which possible matching of patients and controls is done according to outcome.

## Sequential trial design

Sequential trial design does not fix the sample size beforehand and the trial is conducted based on the comparison of two groups. Generally, sequential trial can be completed with a minimum of patients consistent with a statistically significant result, but unfortunately, a sequential trial can only be employed in certain situations.

In sequential trial designs, it is difficult to allow for more than one response variable or for more than two treatments and it will be administratively complex if the trial is multicentre. Sequential trial designs are likely to be of limited use to those therapies where treatment results are generally known too late to limit patient entry.

In commonly used sequential trials, patients enter in matched pairs, one member in each pair receiving (at random) the treatment to be tested and the other a placebo (or alternative treatment). Success or failure of the treatment is determined on each pair of patients sequentially as soon as the results become available and eventually, for each pair, when both treatments are a success or both treatment are a failure, they are discarded from analysis. Usually, a score of +1 is given to an outcome in which tested treatment is a success and placebo alternative treatment a failure, and a score of -1 to an outcome in which placebo or alternative treatment is a success and tested treatment a failure. As the trial proceeds, a cumulative score is kept. It is evident that if tested treatment is markedly superior to alternative treatment, an increasing positive score will be accumulated, whilst an increasing negative score will accumulate in the reverse case. A sequential analysis chart is usually used in the analysis of a clinical trial.

## Single subject experimental designs

Single subject experimental designs (single case designs, n of 1 trial) were developed in the field of psychology and have recently been adapted for clinical research.

Single case designs can evaluate the effectiveness of various specialized acupuncture methods in patients with a variety of individual differences. They are easy to adopt as an exploratory study and their cost is relatively low. Various single subject experimental designs are proposed for clinical trials. In this section, two simple designs are introduced.

A reverse design (AB method) is the simplest n of 1 trial in which baseline data (A) are collected and their stability confirmed before treatment. Then a specific treatment is applied and evaluated by the practitioner. Use of a time series analysis is recommended. Repetitive measurements (ABABAB...) increase the plausibility of results.

In an alternating design, different treatments are repetitively applied in a random order, then the data can be analysed using conventional statistical methods.

However, the latter two techniques are obviously not indicated in the case of acupuncture treatments that have long-lasting or irreversible effects. The results of single subject experimental designs cannot be easily generalized; however, the usefulness of the single subject experimental designs in clinical research on acupuncture should be noted.

## Clinical audit

Clinical audit is a process through which the management of a patient may be improved. The audit cycle is an expansion of a critical approach to the clinical management of patients. Comprehensive data on each patient are required. The aim of the audit is to provide the "best" treatment for a particular patient or illness by continually evaluating the treatment technique against treatment outcome. It is usual to discuss such information within a group of clinicians so that the audit cycle of treatment, critical appraisal and then an improved treatment regimen can be continually developed. The process of a clinical audit creates a positive and supportive environment among acupuncturists. This environment is essential for research development and also allows for the evolution of a research culture and the development of good practice guidelines within acupuncture. The development of "best practice" facilitates the approach required for other research techniques such as RCTs and also acts directly to benefit the patient.

## Acupuncture epidemiology

In the drug evaluation field it has been recognized that information obtained from premarketing clinical trials (phase I, II, III) is imperfect because:

1. the number of patients are limited in the premarketing stage;

2. the drug is used in a range of different conditions after marketing and combined with the other drugs and treatments in complex clinic situations.

Thus, a mechanism called postmarketing surveillance (PMS) has been developed to collect and analyse information in non-trial settings, i.e. general clinical use at primary care level. Originally PMS was designed to collect information about safety but it gradually began to cover effectiveness.

"Pharmaco-epidemiology" is the term used to describe this field. It covers reporting systems, statistical analysis and the necessary drug regulations which allow outcome information to be obtained.

This method can be used in clinic research in countries where acupuncture has legal recognition and in those where it may be recognized in the near future. This methodology could be called "acupuncture epidemiology". The unregulated status of acupuncture in some countries is an obstacle to the development of this area because people who use acupuncture will be reluctant to participate. The official recognition of acupuncture is a prerequisite for the development of acupuncture epidemiology.

"Outcomes research" in relation to acupuncture is synonymous with acupuncture epidemiology. In some countries, information technology can be utilized; computerized databases of health information which cover every aspect of health are a potential source for this research. Medical cards which store all health information for an individual could also be used. Outcomes relate not only to safety, but also, its effectiveness and economic value, i.e. cost-effectiveness. Cohort studies are prospective descriptive studies and can also be utilized in the context of acupuncture epidemiology.

## Medico-anthropological studies

Anthropological research requires an understanding of the social and cultural environment in which acupuncture is practised. This may directly impact on clinical research as it may explain the reasons that, in some countries, there are cultural difficulties in the development of controlled clinical trials and in obtaining informed consent. It also involves cooperation from social scientists and, thus, will allow nongovernmental organizations (NGOs) and government organizations to understand their country's health service requirements and the demands of the population. The socioeconomic and sociopolitical importance of this research is obvious and it must go hand in hand with clinical trials.

# Case report forms

Case report forms (CRFs) are designed to record data on each trial subject during the course of the trial as defined by the protocol. A CRF for each patient in the study must be completed and signed by the investigator and assessor. All the events that happened in the trial should be fully documented, including adverse reactions.

## Data management

The aim of record-keeping and handling of data is to gather information from the study without error in a form that can later be analysed and reported. The investigator and monitor must ensure that the data are of the highest possible quality at the point of collection. A case report form (CRF) for each patient in the study must be completed and signed by the investigator and assessor. The CRF is designed to record data on each trial subject during the course of the trial, as defined by the protocol. The data should be collected by procedures which guarantee preservation, retention and retrieval of information, and allow easy access for verification and audit. The patient's files, CRFs and other sources of primary data must be kept for future reference. Patient data must be handled in a way that maintains confidentiality and yet ensures accuracy. The condition of the patient before treatment, and the response to the treatment, including the observations of the assessor, the feelings of the patient and possible adverse effects, need to be fully documented. All efforts should be made to maintain error-free records.

When subjects are randomized to different groups, the randomization procedure used must be documented.

## Ethics review board

The protocol should be considered by an ethics review board. The board will generally be established at an institutional level, but boards existing at a regional or national level can also be used. The board will be an independent body made up of both medical and non-medical members who are not involved in the experimental activity of evaluation under review. The board will verify that the rights of patients participating in the evaluation are protected and that the trial is justified in both medical and social terms. The board will also consider the suitability of the protocol as it relates to patient selection and patient protection, and the issues of informed consent for patients. However, this board should not promote methodological guidance unless it has appropriate expertise in acupuncture research. The work of the board should be guided by the Helsinki Declaration (see Appendix 2) and other related documents prepared by the individual country or institutions. If beneficial effects are demonstrated for the experimental group, patients allocated to the control group should be offered the possibility of receiving the experimental treatment.

## Statistical analysis

Biostatistical expertise is required when the clinical study is designed, and must continue to be available as data are collected, analysed and prepared for the final report. The misuse of statistical evaluation and abuse of statistical tests is common in all clinical research, particularly in relation to the "t test". Statistical analysis should be made applicable to the nature of the data acquired and the clinical situation in the study. It should always be kept in mind that statistical significance is different from clinical significance. It should not always involve a simple "t test". Every attempt should be made to avoid type II statistical errors and achieve at least an 80% statistical power although 90% would be ideal. Confidence limits should always be stated with the significance values. The value of small group studies can be enhanced by meta-analysis. Failure to complete protocol treatment should be recorded and analysed.

Statistical considerations will govern the number of patients needed to obtain a significant result from the study. The number of patients needed depends on the anticipated difference in the result between the treatment groups in the study. The plan for the statistical analysis to be used at the conclusion of the study must be determined in advance and specified within the protocol. When results are finally analysed, they should be presented in a form that facilitates clinical interpretation.

## Monitoring of studies

A formal procedure for the systematic monitoring of a research project or programme will greatly contribute to its success. Monitoring should be done throughout the period of implementation, and cease only at completion.

Because the therapeutic effect of acupuncture is often observed to continue for a period of time after the completion of a course of treatment, it is recommended that follow-up assessment of subjects should be conducted, particularly in exploratory protocols. The follow-up time may depend on the duration of effects of acupuncture. Inappropriately long or short follow-up times can skew results.

The following elements of the programme or project should be examined: goals, conformity of protocols with goals, progress of the research towards intended goals, and the impact of the research.

The outcome of the study should be evaluated with regard to:

1.      the condition of the patient before treatment;

2.      the progress of the patient's disease stated in terms of both the objective observation made by the investigator or assessor and the patient's own assessment; and

3.      any adverse event that may have occurred during the study.

## Reporting

The chief investigator will be responsible for preparing a final report of the trial which should be provided to the sponsor, the ethics review board, and any other authorities determined by local legislation. The final report is a comprehensive description of the study after its completion including a presentation and evaluation of the results, statistical analyses and a critical ethical, statistical and clinical appraisal. The results of the clinical research conducted on acupuncture should be published in a timely fashion and must include all adverse events. Even studies which fail to demonstrate effectiveness should be published, as selective publication, showing only results that are favourable, will only lead to a form of misconception known as publication bias.

## Implementation

Clear research conclusions have not always been implemented in all fields of medicine, including acupuncture. It is important for clinical researchers to have a clear idea of how their conclusions (both positive and negative) can be implemented and disseminated both within the context of their own health structures and also worldwide.

# Conclusions

The various research methodologies outlined in these guidelines can all contribute some information in the context of research conducted for any purpose. Of all the research methodologies outlined, the randomized controlled (clinical) trials (RCTs) are considered to be the most sophisticated and in many ways have become the "gold standard" for clinical trials in modern clinical research.

There are, however, significant limitations to this approach of RCTs. First, they are often costly, cumbersome, and only incremental answers can be obtained. This is a major drawback in the context of evaluation of whole medical systems such as herbal medicine or acupuncture.

In addition, the RCTs, by definition, eliminate the possible influence of a patient's preference and patient/therapist interaction on the outcome of the treatment. These limitations may be at least partially compensated by carefully designed retrospective and prospective outcome research as described under "Acupuncture epidemiology". Properly planned prospective research is usually superior to retrospective research.

Thus, in the context of acupuncture research, an RCT could be indicated where the purpose of a study is to help improve acupuncture practice, for example, to determine which point combinations are most suited to treat a given condition.

In contrast, acupuncture epidemiology (outcome research) would be indicated where the purpose of research is to evaluate the preventive value of acupuncture or guide patients' choice and health policy.

Finally, while clinical audit and single case studies (n of 1 trial) have a number of inherent limitations, they would be ideal to spur interest in acupuncture research among all researchers and practitioners. Such interest could result in valuable preliminary information generated by an increased positive and critical attitude to ancient traditional statements.

# 6.    USING THE GUIDELINES

These guidelines are intended to facilitate the work of research scientists and clinicians in the field of acupuncture and to provide some reference points for those who contribute to and support clinical studies on acupuncture. The guidelines can also be used by academic institutions. Related appropriate reviews and journals can evaluate reports and articles on the subject. It is hoped that these guidelines will be found general enough to enable institutions in each Member State to modify them to meet their own specific needs. In addition, the guidelines may be useful to health authorities which regulate acupuncture practice and provide indications for acupuncture treatment.

# ANNEXES

# Annex 1

# STRATEGIC APPROACHES TO RANDOMIZED CONTROLLED CLINICAL TRIALS

The neurophysiology of acupuncture has been investigated extensively and reviewed in detail. The principal suggestion is that acupuncture operates largely through neurotransmitters, particularly endorphin-related mechanisms. This argument has been supported almost exclusively by evaluating acupuncture in the context of acute pain within an animal model. These studies demonstrate conclusively that acupuncture's effects are related to the release of a variety of neurotransmitters including natural opiates and, furthermore, that this effect is naloxone-reversible. Basic research work carried out has demonstrated conclusively that any noxious stimulus will result in endorphin release through the neurophysiological mechanism described as diffuse noxious inhibitory control (DNIC). Therefore DNIC represents a nonspecific physiological mechanism which triggers the natural opiate system in both man and experimental animals. There are some studies with human subjects which suggest that acupuncture is not always naloxone-reversible, but they do not fit the general weight of evidence available from animal models. It has been suggested that DNIC plays a relatively minor role in acupuncture analgesia and that other systems, mediated by serotonin and noradrenaline, may be more important.

It is quite probable that chronic pain has different underlying mechanisms from those involved in acute experimental pain in animals. Those working with pain clinics will be only too aware that empirical manipulation of the autonomic system can result in dramatic clinical improvement. In spite of the fact that we do not have a unified theory upon which to explain the mechanism of chronic pain, the empirical evidence available to us would suggest that the autonomic system plays an important, but as yet undefined role, in the complex phenomena involved.

The mechanisms of acupuncture involved in its use as a treatment for addictions almost certainly utilize the endorphin and encephalin systems. There are, however, no detailed studies which define the exact mechanism involved in smoking cessation. Again, it would be reasonable to suggest that the withdrawal symptoms experienced in almost any addictive process may be, at least in part, endorphin-mediated.

The mechanism of acupuncture in internal diseases, such as asthma, irritable bowel, and the treatment of symptoms such as nausea is completely unknown. Acupuncturists have hypothesized that the autonomic nervous system plays an important but as yet ill-defined part in the underlying mechanisms that are involved in the treatment of such internal problems. If we accept that acupuncture might affect the autonomic nervous system in some way, a crucial question now emerges: how is it that needling at some points can affect the autonomic pathways whereas needling at others does not, or does so to a much smaller extent?

It is likely that addictive processes are mediated through neurotransmission which includes the natural opiate systems. Consequently, if we observe clinically that there is no difference between real and sham acupuncture in the treatment of smoking cessation, it is reasonable to suggest that this may be because acupuncture is largely endorphin-mediated in this clinical context. Nonspecific needling may be having as great a clinical effect as specific needling techniques.

In the treatment of nausea however, a non-endorphin mediated mechanism is probably involved. The clinical trial evidence to date suggests that acupuncture has an effect and furthermore that point location is important; needling away from pericardium 6 does not seem to produce as great an effect. It is possible therefore that the theories that underpin traditional medicine relate to an empirical and pragmatic understanding of the autonomic nervous system and its detailed correspondences and effects on the body. If this suggestion is correct, then we would expect that within the treatment of purely internal and non-pain related problems, needling of particular areas, rather than just general stimulation, may be important. Therefore, a sham versus real model may be appropriate in this context.

The final group involves chronic pain. Here there is clear evidence that chronic pain is at least in part mediated through the neurotransmitter, but the empirical evidence suggests that the autonomic system is also important in maintaining a number of chronic pain syndromes. Therefore clinical trials involving acupuncture as a treatment for chronic pain will provide a mixed picture. Sham acupuncture will have some effect through DNIC and will therefore provide a greater effect than that expected from placebo alone. Real acupuncture will utilize the endorphin system but also a putative autonomic response and local trigger-point action, to produce additional effects and therefore an increased clinical response when compared to sham acupuncture. A comparison of acupuncture with placebo in a clinical trial will produce the most clear-cut results when attempting to evaluate acupuncture but point location (real vs sham) may also be important to test the validity of the specific theories concerning point prescription.

# Annex 2

# WORLD MEDICAL ASSOCIATION DECLARATION OF HELSINKI*

Recommendations guiding physicians in biomedical research involving human subjects

Adopted by the 18th World Medical Assembly, Helsinki, Finland, June 1964

and amended by the 29th World Medical Assembly Tokyo, Japan, October 1975

35th World Medical Assembly Venice, Italy, October 1983

and the 41st World Medical Assembly Hong Kong, September 1989

## Introduction

It is the mission of the physician to safeguard the health of the people. His or her knowledge and conscience are dedicated to the fulfilment of this mission.

The Declaration of Geneva of the World Medical Association binds the physician with the words, "The health of my patient will be my first consideration," and the International Code of Medical Ethics declares that, "A physician shall act only in the patient's interest when providing medical care which might have the effect of weakening the physical and mental condition of the patient."

The purpose of biomedical research involving human subjects must be to improve diagnostic, therapeutic and prophylactic procedures and the understanding of the etiology and pathogenesis of disease.

---

* Reprinted by permission from: World Drug Information. Geneva, World Health Organization, 1992 (Vol.6, No.4, pp. 186-188).

In current medical practice most diagnostic, therapeutic or prophylactic procedures involve hazards. This applies especially to biomedical research.

Medical progress is based on research which ultimately must rest in part on experimentation involving human subjects.

In the field of biomedical research, a fundamental distinction must be recognized between medical research in which the aim is essentially diagnostic or therapeutic for a patient, and medical research, the essential object of which is purely scientific and without implying direct diagnostic or therapeutic value to the person subjected to the research.

Special caution must be exercised in the conduct of research which may affect the environment, and the welfare of animals used for research must be respected.

Because it is essential that the results of laboratory experiments be applied to human beings to further scientific knowledge and to help suffering humanity, the World Medical Association has prepared the following recommendations as a guide to every physician in biomedical research involving human subjects. They should be kept under review in the future. It must be stressed that the standards as drafted are only a guide to physicians all over the world. Physicians are not relieved from criminal, civil and ethical responsibilities under the laws of their own countries.

## 1.  Basic principles

1.1  Biomedical research involving human subjects must conform to generally accepted scientific principles and should be based on adequately performed laboratory and animal experimentation and on a thorough knowledge of the scientific literature.

1.2  The design and performance of each experimental procedure involving human subjects should be clearly formulated in an experimental protocol which should be transmitted for consideration, comment and guidance to a specially appointed committee independent of the investigator and the sponsor provided that this independent committee is in conformity with the laws and regulations of the country in which the research experiment is performed.

1.3     Biomedical research involving human subjects should be conducted only by scientifically qualified persons and under the supervision of a clinically competent medical person. The responsibility for the human subject must always rest with a medically qualified person and never rest on the subject of the research, even though the subject has given his or her consent.

1.4     Biomedical research involving human subjects cannot legitimately be carried out unless the importance of the objective is in proportion to the inherent risk to the subject.

1.5     Every biomedical research project involving human subjects should be preceded by careful assessment of predictable risks in comparison with foreseeable benefits to the subject or to others. Concern for the interests of the subject must always prevail over the interests of science and society.

1.6     The right of the research subject to safeguard his or her integrity must always be respected. Every precaution should be taken to respect the privacy of the subject and to minimize the impact of the study on the subject's physical and mental integrity and on the personality of the subject.

1.7     Physicians should abstain from engaging in research projects involving human subjects unless they are satisfied that the hazards involved are believed to be predictable. Physicians should cease any investigation if the hazards are found to outweigh the potential benefits.

1.8     In publication of the results of his or her research, the physician is obliged to preserve the accuracy of the results. Reports of experimentation not in accordance with the principles laid down in this Declaration should not be accepted for publication.

1.9     In any research on human beings, each potential subject must be adequately informed of the aims, methods, anticipated benefits and potential hazards of the study and the discomfort it may entail. He or she should be informed that he or she is at liberty to abstain from participation in the study and that he or she is free to withdraw his or her consent to participation at any time. The physician should then obtain the subject's freely-given informed consent, preferably in writing.

1.10    When obtaining informed consent for the research project, the physician should be particularly cautious if the subject is in a dependent relationship to him or her or may consent under duress. In that case, the informed consent should be obtained by a physician who is not engaged in the investigation and who is completely independent of this official relationship.

1.11    In case of legal incompetence, informed consent should be obtained from the legal guardian in accordance with national legislation. Where physical or mental incapacity makes it impossible to obtain informed consent, or when the subject is a minor, permission from the responsible relative replaces that of the subject in accordance with national legislation.

Whenever the minor child is in fact able to give a consent, the minor's consent must be obtained in addition to the consent of the minor's legal guardian.

1.12    The research protocol should always contain a statement of the ethical considerations involved and should indicate that the principles enunciated in the present Declaration are complied with.

## 2.    Medical research combined with professional care (Clinical research)

2.1    In the treatment of the sick person, the physician must be free to use a new diagnostic and therapeutic measure, if in his or her judgement it offers hope of saving life, reestablishing health or alleviating suffering.

2.2    The potential benefits, hazards and discomfort of a new method should be weighed against the advantages of the best current diagnostic and therapeutic methods.

2.3    In any medical study, every patient - including those of a control group, if any - should be assured of the best proven diagnostic and therapeutic method.

2.4    The refusal of the patient to participate in a study must never interfere with the physician-patient relationship.

2.5    If the physician considers it essential not to obtain informed consent, the specific reasons for this proposal should be stated in the experimental protocol for transmission to the independent committee (1, 2).

2.6    The physician can combine medical research with professional care, the objective being the acquisition of new medical knowledge, only to the extent that medical research is justified by its potential diagnostic or therapeutic value for the patient.

## 3.   Non-therapeutic biomedical research involving human subjects

### (Non-clinical biomedical research)

3.1    In the purely scientific application of medical research carried out on a human being, it is the duty of the physician to remain the protector of the life and health of that person on whom biomedical research is being carried out.

3.2    The subjects should be volunteers - either health persons or patients for whom the experimental design is not related to the patient's illness.

3.3    The investigator or the investigating team should discontinue the research if in his/her or their judgment it may, if continued, be harmful to the individual.

3.4    In research on man, the interest of science and society should never take precedence over considerations related to the well-being of the subject.

# Annex 3

# REPORT OF THE WORKING GROUP ON CLINICAL RESEARCH METHODOLOGY FOR ACUPUNCTURE AOMORI, JAPAN, 1-4 JUNE 1994

## Summary

The Working Group on Clinical Research Methodology for Acupuncture met in Aomori, Japan, from 1 to 4 June 1994. The main objective of the meeting was to develop guidelines for clinical research on acupuncture and to make recommendations on further collaboration and activity on clinical research of acupuncture.

The meeting was attended by 12 members from six Member States, one secretariat staff from the WHO Regional Office for the Western Pacific and three observers from Japan.

Dr Sung-Keel Kang was elected Chairman, Dr K. Segami, Vice-Chairman and Dr Daniel Eskinazi, Rapporteur. Dr S.T. Han, WHO's Regional Director for the Western Pacific, delivered a speech during the closing ceremony.

The members presented their papers to review the current status of clinical research on acupuncture. The drafts of guidelines for clinical research on acupuncture were discussed extensively. The issues covered during the discussion included: the definition of terms used in the guidelines; organization of clinical research on acupuncture; ethical problems involved in the process of clinical research; research methods; and concepts expressed in the guidelines.

In the course of these discussions, the Working Group developed the guidelines for clinical research on acupuncture and made recommendations for promoting the dissemination of the guidelines. A summary of these recommendations follows:

1.  Each interested Member State should develop a national programme that will be proactive and designed to make available: (a) safe and effective acupuncture through clinical research studies; and (b) unbiased information to the public to help guide patients' preferences.

2.  Interested Member States should specify a centre or centres of excellence in order to coordinate their country's programmes.

3.  Research education of interested acupuncturists and other health professionals should form an essential first step in developing a research culture within each Member State through: (a) dissemination of the guidelines for clinical research on acupuncture; (b) publication of the guidelines in book form, multilingually; and (c) development of a programme of clinical research methodology workshops in interested Member States based on the guidelines.

4.  Each Member State should consider the ethical problems involved in the process of clinical research.

5.  Information exchange should be assured among all interested parties.

6.  Standard acupuncture nomenclature should be used (wherever possible) in all clinical research projects.

7.  Detailed research strategies in relation to disease-oriented research proposals should be developed.

8.  Cooperation between acupuncturists and other health care providers should be fostered.

9.  The practice of acupuncture should receive an introduction in the medical education system.

10.	The Working Group realizes that WHO may not have the necessary resources to directly implement all the recommendations outlined above. However, it is recommended that WHO should play the leading and coordinating role, and involve appropriate organizations and associations in implementing these recommendations.

# 1.	Introduction

Acupuncture has been practised in China for more than 2500 years. It was introduced to neighbouring countries like Japan, the Republic of Korea and Viet Nam early in the 6th century. Because of the wide indication of its therapeutic properties, the simplicity of its application, and its low cost and rapid results for treatment of many disorders, acupuncture has spread worldwide during the last 20 years.

Following the growing interest in acupuncture, clinical research on its effectiveness has been carried out by acupuncturists, clinicians and other researchers, particularly in east Asia. However, it is noted that the quality of research still varies considerably, and some difficulty in applying common scientific principles to clinical research on acupuncture has been experienced by many researchers.

In 1987, during its thirty-eighth session, the WHO Regional Committee for the Western Pacific adopted a resolution on traditional medicine which urged Member States to undertake research to evaluate the safety and efficacy of traditional medicine, based on the concepts of both modern and traditional medicines. The Scientific Group on Acupuncture which met in October 1989 in Geneva, recommended that WHO should play a role in consolidating guidelines on research methodology to ensure the comparability of results.

The WHO Regional Office for the Western Pacific (WHO/WPRO) has played an important role in the development of standard terminology and technology on traditional medicine, including acupuncture. The Working Group on Clinical Research Methodology for Acupuncture was constituted by the WHO Regional Office for the Western Pacific to review and finalize the Guidelines for Clinical Research on Acupuncture prepared by the Traditional Medicine Unit in WHO/WPRO. The Guidelines provide the basic principles and standards for preparing, conducting and evaluating clinical research on acupuncture. The Working Group met in Aomori, Japan from 1 to 4 June 1994.

## 1.1 Objectives

The objectives of the meeting were as follows:

1. to review the current status of clinical research on acupuncture in the Region;

2. to discuss the methodology used for clinical research on acupuncture;

3. to review and finalize the guidelines for clinical research on acupuncture; and

4. to make recommendations on further collaboration and activities in the field of research on acupuncture.

## 1.2 Participants

The Working Group is composed of 12 temporary advisers and one member of the WHO Secretariat. Three observers from Japan also attended the meeting. The list of participants is shown in Annex 4.

## 1.3 Organization

Professor Sung-Keel Kang and Dr K. Segami were elected Chairman and Vice-Chairman of the Working Group. Dr Daniel Eskinazi was elected Rapporteur.

## 1.4 Opening ceremony

Owing to a previous commitment, Dr S.T. Han, Regional Director of the WHO Regional Office for the Western Pacific, was not able to attend the opening ceremony.

Dr Chen Ken, Medical Officer for Traditional Medicine, delivered the speech on behalf of Dr Han. During his speech, Dr Han pointed out that acupuncture has been widely recognized as a valuable and readily available means of health care and is effective, requiring only simple equipment and inexpensive medical techniques. However, he indicated that a lack of well-designed and conducted research on acupuncture has affected its acceptance. He reminded the Working Group that WHO considered research on acupuncture to be essential and the main purpose of WHO in developing guidelines for clinical research on acupuncture was to guide researchers in designing and conducting clinical research to improve the quality of research activities. He insisted that the criteria and theories of oriental philosophy reflected in acupuncture should be respected, and that the promotion of clinical research did not mean that acupuncture's efficacy should be evaluated only according to the methodology used by modern medicine. He noted that the Working Group had the responsibility to finalize the first guidelines in the Region to be applied to clinical research on acupuncture.

During the opening ceremony, Mr Masaya Kitamura, Governor of Aomori Prefecture, Dr Hiroyuki Doi, Deputy Director, International Affairs Division of the Ministry of Health and Welfare, Japan and Dr Takayoshi Harada, Chairman of Aomori Medical Association, gave their welcome speeches.

# 2. Proceedings

## 2.1 Presentation

The current status of clinical research on acupuncture and the methodology used for clinical evaluation of acupuncture were outlined in the working papers prepared by the members of the Working Group. The papers submitted are summarized below.

Dr Chen Ken indicated that WHO is aware of the value of acupuncture for maintaining health, and its possible potential contribution to WHO's goal of health for all. In June 1977, WHO organized an Interregional Seminar on Acupuncture Moxibustion and Acupuncture Anaesthesia in Beijing, China. In 1985 and 1987, two resolutions on traditional medicine were adopted by the Regional Committee for the Western Pacific, which formed the policy basis and programme direction of traditional medicine. After summarizing WHO's programme activities in the field of acupuncture, he introduced the procedure of preparation of draft guidelines. The guidelines drafted by WPRO, were sent out to 20 experts from different countries both within and outside the Region, for comments. Based on the comments received by the Regional Office, the guidelines were revised several times. The Working Group was asked to discuss and finalize the guidelines.

Dr Eskinazi, Deputy Director, Office of Alternative Medicine, National Institute of Health (NIH), United States of America, informed the group that the NIH Office of Alternative Medicine (OAM) was created by the US Congress in October 1991 and is a permanent part of the NIH structure. It is currently located in the Office of the Director. Its mission is to evaluate any form of alternative medicine. Acupuncture is one of these "alternative medicines". Thus far, OAM has taken essentially two approaches to research in acupuncture. First, it has funded a few research grants dealing with protocols evaluating the efficacy of acupuncture in dealing with specific medical conditions. Second, it has organized a conference with the cooperation of the Food and Drug Administration (FDA). The purpose of the conference was to present a thorough analysis of the acupuncture scientific literature to help FDA re-evaluate regulations. This re-evaluation may have a significant impact on the acceptance and patterns of acupuncture use in the United States.

Professor S.K. Kang, College of Oriental Medicine, Kyung Hee University, Republic of Korea and Dr Y.S. Kim, Department of Acupuncture and Moxibustion, Kyung Hee University, Republic of Korea, summarized the clinical research on acupuncture covered in the Republic of Korea. There are a number of clinical acupuncture reports detailing excellent improvements; however, they have not been conducted by controlled studies owing to their cultural background. Most of the patients do not want to be experimental subjects. Therefore, many of the acupuncture studies have been conducted by animal experimental trials in the Republic of Korea. Currently, many doctors are interested in the clinical research methodology for acupuncture. By reviewing and analysing clinical research papers taken from MEDLINE, the general issues in acupuncture research in the Republic of Korea may be divided into three parts: selection of point, mode of stimulation and determination of placebo group for acupuncture. It is recommended that the compromised form of control-placebo for acupuncture is carried on in clinical trials.

Dr Lewith, The Centre for the Study of Complementary Medicine, United Kingdom, re-examined the three areas which have encompassed the major part of clinical research into acupuncture: chronic pain, addiction (in particular smoking cessation), and the treatment of nausea and vomiting. Clarification of the findings, and of the different control conditions that have been used, suggests that point location is an important variable in the treatment of chronic pain and nausea, but not of addiction. These observations can be explained by postulating that different underlying mechanisms are involved in the treatment of different conditions: addictions may be mediated purely by opioid peptides, nausea by the autonomic system and a combination of both may be involved in chronic pain, together with local trigger point action. A hypothesis is presented which suggests that the closer one gets to a purely endorphin-mediated effect, the less relevant it is to think in terms of point location and the more misleading a real versus sham acupuncture model is in the context of a clinical trial. The hypothesis is necessarily speculative but it does provide a coherent theoretical framework which integrates neurophysiology, our current knowledge of clinical trials, and some aspects of traditional Chinese medicine.

Professor Meng Xian Kun, Director, Acupuncture Department, Dong Zhi Men Hospital, China, described the most commonly-used clinical research methods for acupuncture in China. They are: (1) clinical observation; (2) clinical experiment; and (3) summing-up of the clinical experience of famous acupuncturists. Clinical observation is still the dominant method employed in China, although, the academic value of observational studies varies greatly. He suggested that careful consideration should be given to selection of research topics, selection of cases, use of control groups, randomization, use of blind technique, application of treatment, evaluation of outcome and statistical analysis.

Dr K. Nishijo, Professor, Department of Acupuncture, Tsukuba College of Medical Technology and Nursing, Japan; Dr K. Segami, Executive Director and in charge of Deputy Director-General, Department of Health and Medical Services and Environmental Control, the Government of Aomori, Japan; Dr T. Shichido, Head, Information and Evaluation Group, Research Committee, Scientific Group, Society of Acupuncture, Japan and Dr K. Tsutani, Associate Professor, Department of Clinical Pharmacology, Division of Information and Science, Medical Research Institute, Tokyo Medical and Dental University, Japan, reviewed two bibliometrical studies on acupuncture and analysis of the controlled studies of acupuncture. A MEDLINE search reveals that a sharp increase of the number of acupuncture papers occurred in the early 1970s, and that about 300 papers are produced annually. Altogether, 3000 papers on acupuncture are found in MEDLINE, of which 30% are from China, 20% from the former Soviet Union, 10% from the United States, 10% from the United Kingdom, 3% from Germany and 2% from Japan. However, biased inclusion of journals in MEDLINE was noted. For instance, no journals on acupuncture and Japanese oriental medicine are indexed there. Japan Centra Revuo Medicine was searched in its CD-ROM format. About 2000 papers were found from 1987 to 1993, or an average of 300 papers annually. Most of the papers are on human beings, and published in journals of acupuncture or Japanese oriental medicine, but few are controlled studies. Most of them are descriptive studies, some combining laboratory evaluation, mechanism of action, treatment technique, discussions on meridian and discussions in clinics. A manual search revealed that 13 controlled trials have been conducted in Japan since 1966. There are, however, several problems in design, sample size, description of randomization, blinding and control, handling of drop-out cases and incorrect statistical analysis and interpretation (i.e. inappropriate conclusions in the light of data reported).

Professor Nguyen Tai Thu, Director, National Institute of Acupuncture, Viet Nam, introduced experiences in clinical use and research on acupuncture. During the past 30 years, acupuncture has been used to treat not only common diseases but also difficult cases. Acupuncture analgesia has been carried out for about 28 000 patients undergoing surgery.

Professor Zhuang Ding, Institute of Acupuncture and Moxibustion, China Academy of Traditional Medicine, China, reviewed the organization of clinical research on acupuncture in China, its current status and problems encountered during clinical research on acupuncture. In the last 40 years, a great deal of work has been done on clinical research on acupuncture in China and more than 20 000 articles have been published in various journals or presented at academic meetings. However, some researchers lack strict scientific training, and this can be identified in their reports. In some research reports, the observed patients were outpatients, who may still have been receiving other kinds of medical treatment without a control on them.  Thus the observed therapeutic result was achieved through complicated treatment, not acupuncture alone.  In other research, when the treating course lasted for several months, the number of patients who continued treatment was quite different from the number at the beginning.  In another report, curative effect statistics included only those who continued their treatment, and not those who failed.  Consequently, the statistics did not meet the requirements of medical statistics, although the survey was carried out in a statistical way.  The high curative rate was therefore not solely the result of acupuncture.

## 2.2    Discussion

The draft guidelines prepared by WPRO were used as the basic document for discussion.

### 2.2.1 Overview

The discussion was devoted to concepts expressed in the guidelines and to creating a sample outline of the guidelines.

In terms of concepts, it was agreed that no simple and methodological approach could cover all acupuncture research.  Instead, methodologies need to be tailored to the questions asked.  The notions of simple case prospective studies as well as that of outcome research were introduced and discussed.  The purposes of conducting research for guiding physicians' choices on the one hand and patients' choices (which would also be reflected by choice due to ethnic background) on the other, were also discussed.  It became clear that these two different demands could be best met by randomized controlled trials and by outcome research respectively.

It was agreed that it would be helpful to be very explicit and that a glossary should be included.  In this context, the notion of randomization of sampling versus that of allocation was clarified.

After briefly debating whether a specific example (e.g. asthma) should be discussed, it was decided that only statements not referring to specific conditions should be made in the guidelines.  However, examples should be randomly chosen to illustrate the various points covered in the final document.

Before closing the session, a tentative structure was adopted as a working model for the guidelines. This would include:

1.　　background on acupuncture;

2.　　the purpose of research and what constitutes research;

3.　　general considerations; and

4.　　research methodologies.

## 2.2.2 Specific issues

1.　　Research methods

This group considered the following issues in relation to research methodology:

    a.　Existing data on acupuncture have a cultural bias but form the essential first step of any research project.

    b.　Descriptive research outlines the uncontrolled effects of acupuncture with respect to:

        -　traditional medicinal systems;

        -　cultural aspects of each country's health provision;

        -　the process or techniques of the acupuncture utilized; and

        -　outcomes (objective and subjective).

    c.　A clinical trial (CT) is one of the clinical research methods available. A clinical trial consists of four elements:

        (i) it is carried out on human beings;

        (ii) it has an evaluation purpose (efficacy and safety);

        (iii) it is conducted intensively; and

        (iv) it is a scientific experiment.

d.  Randomized controlled clinical trials (RCTs) provide detailed outcome information.  The problems and difficulties in relation to RCTs involving acupuncture are outlined by the group.

e.  Outcome research analyses data retrospectively in relation to the clinical effects and cost-effectiveness of acupuncture with respect to other "possibly conventional" treatments.

f.  Single case studies are analyses carried out prospectively on the effects of a planned treatment regimen on one individual.

New research strategies also need to be considered based on a realistic assessment of the cost and cultural and political environment in which health care operates.  These include:

-   pragmatic research that compares outcomes and cases of different treatment packages (conventional and traditional);

-   development research ("fix, maintain, contain") that allows us to develop a better understanding of cost and cost-effectiveness.

2.      Outcome measurements in relation to research

The group agreed that research is needed to provide information about one or more of the following points:

a.  effectiveness;

b.  cost-effectiveness;

c.  efficacy;

d.  preventive effects of acupuncture;

e.  safety;

f.  utility; and

g.  benefit.

Particular attention needs to be paid to:

    a.  cultural and ethnic factors that may promote research;

    b.  outcome measures designed to answer the questions raised by the hypothesis being tested;

    c.  statistical techniques relevant to the disease studied;

    d.  the assumptions made within a particular system of traditional medicine; and

    e.  the process of random allocation in relation to patient choice and outcome.

3.      Terminology

Proper understanding of terminology in clinical research such as randomization, blindness, placebo, validity, reliability and generalizability is most important in discussions on sound development of clinical research methodology for acupuncture.

The group agreed that a glossary with working definitions would be included in the Guidelines.

4.      Ethical issues

Although fundamental human rights are fully recognized by the Working Group and should be respected in clinical research, including acupuncture research, there are different national interpretations in countries where acupuncture is officially recognized and those where acupuncture is not fully recognized.

In those countries where acupuncture has a long history, acupuncture practitioners as well as patients have a cultural barrier accepting the concept of ethical issues developed in the west, such as informed consent. In other countries where acupuncture is not yet recognized, to conduct clinical trial without informed consent is an abuse of human rights.

## 2.3    Field visit

The members of the Working Group visited Aomori Oriental Medical Hospital and the library affiliated with the hospital.

## 2.4    Closing ceremony

Dr S.T. Han, Regional Director of the WHO Regional Office for the Western Pacific, pointed out in his closing remarks
that this was the first attempt to produce research guidelines for acupuncture, and it would enhance scientific research on acupuncture not only in the Western Pacific Region but other parts of the world as well. He indicated that WHO supports scientific research on acupuncture; however, the experience obtained by its use over many years should not be ignored.  He noted that the group had fulfilled the objectives of the Meeting and he assured the group that the Regional Office would continue its leading role in the promotion of the proper use of acupuncture.

On behalf of all participants, Dr Eskinazi acknowledged the effort and support of the WHO Regional Office for the Western Pacific in holding the Working Group Meeting and in developing the Guidelines for Clinical Research on Acupuncture.

# 3.    Conclusions and recommendations

## 3.1    Conclusions

3.1.1    The Guidelines for Clinical Research on Acupuncture were finalized.  The Working Group successfully fulfilled the task assigned to it.

3.1.2    As a valid and effective health care approach, acupuncture should be accepted by health service systems, even though the Working Group recognizes that further clinical research is required.

3.1.3   The consensus reached by the Working Group on social, cultural and ethical considerations and basic principles, methodologies used in clinical research on acupuncture and other related issues, are set out in the Guidelines for Clinical Research on Acupuncture. The recommendations of the Working Group are outlined below.

## 3.2   Recommendations

It is essential to develop a worldwide research culture through which acupuncture can be evaluated, thus providing the background for all the detailed recommendations within this report. The advent of a research-led decision-making process will be achieved by a process of continued education and development. It is recognized that this ideal will not occur immediately but we believe that a number of simple recommendations can be implemented which will, in time, begin this process. Further review of these recommendations will be required over a certain time.

3.2.1   Each interested Member State should develop a national programme that will be proactive and designed to make available:

1. acupuncture where it has been shown to be safe and effective through appropriate clinical research studies; and

2. unbiased information to the public to help guide patients' preferences.

3.2.2   It is recommended that interested Member States specify a centre or centres of excellence to coordinate their country's programmes.

3.2.3   The research education of interested acupuncturists and other health professionals would form an essential first step in developing a research culture within each Member State. In order to implement this general principle, a number of specific activities are recommended:

1. the widespread dissemination of the Guidelines for Clinical Research on Acupuncture. This can be effected by publication of hard copy, electronic publication, the active assistance of acupuncture associations on a worldwide basis and the active participation of medical schools and medical research establishments;

2. the publication of the Guidelines in book form, in various languages; and

3. the development of a programme of clinical research methodology workshops based on the Guidelines in interested Member States. The workshops should be designed to initiate a research culture that is practical and should be realistically tailored to the audience and also relevant to the local health care system. The effectiveness of the workshops will ultimately be reflected in the quality of published research.

3.2.4 The group recommends that each Member State should consider the ethical problems involved in the process of clinical research. Particular attention should be paid to patient safety, confidentiality, informed consent, and overall care as it applies in the cultural context of each Member State. Further studies should be conducted in relation to the ethical issues involved in clinical research on acupuncture. Consideration should be given to the different value systems that are involved in human rights such as social, cultural and historical issues.

3.2.5 Information is now frequently exchanged worldwide. Effective clinical research requires an international database of published research. The development of a unified and effective research database is essential. All too often, databases are underused. Therefore, an active programme of promotion and education must go hand-in-hand with database investment and development. Duplication of efforts should be avoided. Institutions such as the National Institute of Health and the databases available in the Institute of Information in the China Academy of Traditional Chinese Medicine, supported by WHO, should coordinate their efforts to make research databases available on a worldwide basis.

3.2.6 Standard acupuncture nomenclature should be used (wherever possible) in all clinical research projects. Further promotional activity in relation to the standardization of acupuncture technology and point location is recommended.

3.2.7 Detailed research strategies in relation to disease-oriented research proposals should be developed. This will require specific workshops that focus on particular illnesses defined by clear conventional or traditional diagnoses.

3.2.8 To foster cooperation between acupuncturists and other health care providers.

3.2.9 The group recommends the practice of acupuncture in the medical education system. This may involve a simple basic introduction as a first step that just outlines its mechanism, uses and abuses.

3.2.10 The Working Group realizes that WHO may not have the necessary resources to directly implement all the recommendations outlined above. However, it is recommended that WHO play a leadership and coordinating role, and involve appropriate organizations and associations in implementing these recommendations.

# Annex 4

# LIST OF MEMBERS, OBSERVERS AND SECRETARIAT OF THE WORKING GROUP ON CLINICAL RESEARCH METHODOLOGY FOR ACUPUNCTURE AOMORI, JAPAN 1-4 JUNE 1994

## 1.    Members

Dr Daniel Eskinazi
Deputy Director
Office of the Alternative Medicine
National Institute of Health
Bethesda, Maryland 20892
United States of America

Professor Sung-Keel Kang
Professor
Department of Acupuncture
and Moxibustion
College of Oriental Medicine
Kyung Hee University
Seoul, 130-702
Republic of Korea

Dr Yong-Suk Kim
Clinical Researcher
Hospital of Oriental Medicine
Kyung Hee University
Seoul 130-702
Republic of Korea

Professor Le The Trung
Member of the National Council of
Scientific and Technological Policies
Permanent Member of Executive Council
of the Vietnamese Association of
Traditional Medicine
Hanoi, Viet Nam

Dr George Lewith
Centre for the Study
of Complementary Medicine
51 Bedford Place, Southampton
Hampshire S01 2DG
United Kingdom

Professor Meng Xian Kun
Professor of Medicine
Director
Acupuncture Department
Dong Zhi Men Hospital
Beijing University of
Traditional Chinese Medicine
Beijing
China

Professor Nguyen Tai Thu
Director, National Institute
of Acupuncture
Hanoi
Viet Nam

Dr Kazushi Nishijo
Professor
Department of Acupuncture
Tsukuba College of Medicinal
Technology and Nursing
University of Tsukuba
Tokyo
Japan

Dr K. Segami
Executive Director and in-charge
of Deputy Director-General,
Department of Health and
Medical Services and
Environmental Science of
Aomori Prefectural Government
Aomori
Japan

Dr Toshiyuki Shichido
Head
Information and
Evaluation Group (IEG)
Research Committee,
Scientific Department,
Japan Society of Acupuncture
Tokyo
Japan

Dr K. Tsutani
Associate Professor
Department of Clinical Pharmacology
Division of Information Medicine
Medical Research Institute
Tokyo Medical and Dental University
Tokyo
Japan

Dr Zhuang Ding
Professor of Physiology
Institute of Acupuncture
China Academy of Traditional
Chinese Medicine
Beijing
China

## 2. Observers

Dr Kenji Kawakita
Professor
Department of Physiology
Meiji College of Oriental Medicine
Kyoto
Japan

Dr Yukio Kurosu
Vice-President
Japan Society of Acupuncture
Tokyo
Japan

Dr Shozho Hosina
President
Aomori Acupuncture Association
President
Tohoku Acupuncture Society
Towada-shi
Japan

## 3. Secretariat

Dr Chen Ken
Medical Officer
Traditional Medicine
World Health Organization
for the Western Pacific Region
Manila
Philippines

# BIBLIOGRAPHY


1.  Proposed WHO guidelines for good clinical practice (GCP) for trials on pharmaceutical products. WHO drug information, 1992; 6(4): 170-188.

2.  Research Guidelines for Evaluating the Safety and Efficacy of Herbal Medicines, World Health Organization, Regional Office for the Western Pacific, Manila, 1993.

3.  Health Research Methodology. A Guide for Training in Research Methods, WHO Regional Office for the Western Pacific, Manila, 1992.

4.  International Ethical Guidelines of Biomedical Research Involving Human Subjects CIOMS. Geneva 1993.

5.  Bailar, J.C. IV and Mosteller, F., Medical Uses of Statistics, Second Edition, NZJM Books, 1992.

6.  Meinert, C.L., Clinical Trials - Design, Conduct and Analysis. Oxford University Press, New York/Oxford, 1976.

7.  Sackett, D.L., Clinical Epidemiology, A Basic Science for Clinical Medicine, Second Edition, Little, Brown and Company. Boston/ Toronto/London, 1991.

8.  Lewith, G. and Aldridge, D., Clinical Research Methodology for Complementary Therapies, Hodder & Stoughton, 1993.

9.  Daly, L.E. et al. Interpretation and Uses of Medical Statistics, Fourth Edition, Blackwell Scientific Publications, Oxford, 1991.

10. Fletcher, R.H. et al. Clinical epidemiology - the essentials. Williams & Wilkins, Baltimore, 1988.

11.	김정순 (Jung-Soon Kim): 疫學原論 4版 (Principle of Clinical Epidemiology, 4th edition), 新光出版社 (Shinkwang Publishing Company), Seoul, 1993.

12.	김정혜 (Jung-Hye Kim): 疫學 및 傳染病管理 (Epidemiology and Management of Infectious Diseases), 青丘出版社 (Chungku Publishing Company), Seoul, 1993.

13.	佐久問昭 (Sakuma, Akira): 藥效評價 (Drug Evaluation), 1 and 2, Tokyo University Press, Tokyo, 1977 and 1981.

14.	砂原茂一 (Sunahara, Shigeichi): 臨床醫學研究序説 (Introduction of Clinical Research Methodology and Ethics), Igakushain, Tokyo, 1988.

15.	王家良 (Wang Jialiang): 临床流行病学，临床科研，设计，衡量与评价(Clinical Epidemiology: Clinical Research Design, Measurement and Evaluation), 上海科技出版社, Shanghai Science and Technology Publication House, Shanghai, 1990.

16.	金丕焕 (Jin Pihuan): 医学统计方法 (Methodology for Medical Statistics), 上海医科大学出版社, Shanghai Medical University Publication House, Shanghai, 1993.

17.	曹家琪 Cao Jiaqui): 临床医学研究方法学 (Methodology for Clinical Research), 北京医科大学，北京协和医科大学联合出版， Beijing Medical University and Peking Union Medical University Publication House, Beijing, 1993.